BABAL

SANTERÍA AND THE
LORD OF PESTILENCE

BY BABA RAUL CANIZARES
& ABURO ERIC LERNER

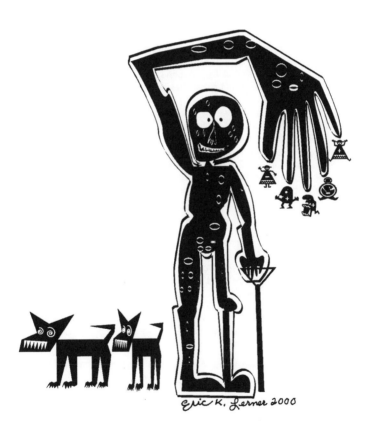

Eric K. Lerner 2000

ORIGINAL PUBLICATIONS
PLAINVIEW, NEW YORK

BABALÚ AYÉ
SANTERÍA AND THE LORD OF PESTILENCE
By Baba Raul Canizares
and Aburo Eric Lerner

ISBN: 0-942272-62-5

FIRST EDITION
First Printing 2000

Cover art by Raul Canizares
Interior illustrations by Raul Canizares
Title Page Illustration by Eric Lerner

Original Publications
P.O. Box 236
Old Bethpage, New York 11804-0236
(516) 454-6809

Printed in the United States of America

1

INTRODUCTION

SONPONNA. IT IS NOT GOOD OF YOU NOT TO SPARE ME!
BUT IF YOU WANT TO CARRY MY LOAD,
LET ME FOLLOW YOU TO YOUR HOME BY THE RIVER.
JINGLING HORSEMAN IN A CLOUD OF DUST,
CARRY ME TO YOUR HOME IN THE BUSH,
HEAVENLY TORMENTOR, HOLD ME. HOLD ME IN YOUR ARM.[1]

It's mid-December. The sky glows eerily red, the unpaved roads leading from the city of Havana to the only leprosarium left in Cuba at the little township of El Rincón are packed. These are pilgrims, but most outsiders would be hard pressed to recognize them as such. Fellini would have a field day filming the scenes that unfold as one moves from one point to the next along the bizarre journey. It is my first time participating in a defining act of Cuban piety: walking from wherever it is you live to the shrine of St. Lazarus. I dare say about 25% of the pilgrims are strict Catholics, the rest belonging to one or more of the four great African-derived religions of Cuba: Santeria, Palo, Abakuá, and Arará. I was only seven and, luckily, our home was a mere thirty miles away from El Rincón. Those coming from Oriente province had to walk--or crawl, or worse--over seven hundred miles!

As a kid, I enjoy all of it, the carnival atmosphere, the vendors selling pork sandwiches drenched in fried onions, the loudspeakers playing the same song, *"Hasta El Rincón a pie!"* which loosely translated means *"To El Rincón or bust!"* A young man joins Mother, Andres (the family servant who also functioned as one of our Santeria elders) and me. He is from Oriente, he says in the sing-song accent of that part of our island, and he promised *el viejo Lazaro* to walk barefoot to his shrine if he gave his mother one more year to live. Apparently Old Man Lazaro came through, because the lad showed his bare feet to us, cracked and bleeding. I'm happy Andres came along, for after ten miles the soles of my feet begin to burn and I welcome being carried on Andres' muscular shoulders.

Like us, many have traveled a long distance to the tiny village that lives off the income provided by this yearly pilgrimage. The crimson strangeness of the night is accentuated by thousands of votives. A young woman in a wheelchair is pushed along by her family. Her grandmother smooths her damp wiry hair and wails, clutching a chromolith of San Lazaro to her breast. A little way down the road, a nearly naked man sprawls across the ground as companions stand on his barrel chest and pour candle wax on him in a testament to endurance. Some drag themselves along the ground with rocks tied to their feet. Others wear Sunday finery. Little girls with flowers braided in their hair share the path with scrawny men in rags. Odors of flowers, perfume, sweat and roadside barbecues mingle in a not unpleasant mix that makes the experience special.

A massive confluence of humanity converges each December 17th on the chapel of San Lazaro at the leprosarium. The statue of the old man on crutches, suffering from painful boils and having only two little dogs for company is so bedecked in gold that only his face is visible. Prominent among the gold gifts visible behind the glass enclosure where the statue stands is the solid gold and diamond Rolex Presidente that Fulgencio Batista gave as proof of his gratitude to San Lazaro for saving the life of his cancer-stricken wife. Batista had been Cuba's dictator before Fidel Castro defeated him in 1959.

Technically speaking, neither the strict Roman Catholics nor the Afro-Cuban practitioners come to honor the Lazarus that the chapel is named for. The "leper" Lazarus appears in the Bible as a component in a parable Jesus said about a rich man and a poor man. As is well known, parables are allegorical tales intended to clarify and illustrate certain points. The Lazarus of the parable, therefore, is not recognized by the Catholic Church as a real person. Other saints named Lazarus, however, do exist, including Bishop Lazarus, for whom the chapel is named. His statue is there, also, in the main altar, lonely and without a single piece of gold. So why does the Catholic Church allow the veneration of an imaginary saint? The official explanation is that the leper Lazarus "might" have existed, and that because of the millions of people who venerate him, he has become a "saint by acclamation." The majority of people who go to honor the old man, however, are not even honoring the parable Lazarus, but an ancient African god named Babalu Aye.[2]

Babalu Aye means "father of the earth." In Africa, it is a praise name used to describe Sonponna, the Orisha of small pox. As evidenced by his annual pilgrimage, he is among the most important and beloved deities in Cuban Santeria. The most tenderly loved of the Orisha in Cuba, he is a feared deity in Africa. This may be because it is he who both afflicts people with illness and heals them. "O dá éé. O dá e," "He cuts you many times. He cures you."[3] says a popular refrain in his Cuban praise songs. In Africa, some believe that to speak his true name is to invite pestilence.

Babalu Aye historically is associated with many forms of pestilence, particularly smallpox, leprosy, and, most recently, AIDS. Babalu's worship has long involved the control of contagion. E. Bolaji Idowu in his seminal work *Olodumare God in Yoruba Belief* portrayed the role of his priests. They took charge of the bodies of those who died from infectious disease. As payment, they would frequently demand all of the deceased's personal effects which were burned as an offering. This curbed transmission. Bolaji and others suggest they would also retain some of the dead's belongings and even their blood and body parts to use them to afflict illness and death. However, this is an interpretation of mostly Christian clerics who demonized orisha worshippers. What is certain is that these priests had knowledge of vaccination and would inoculate cult members against small pox by inserting bits of infected material in incisions. They've long known how to live with disease.

Babalu gives his devotees means to survive. Ulli Beier, a seasoned scholar and poet of Yoruba culture, elaborates on this point:

> Sakpata [Babalu] is the god of suffering. He teaches his
> worshippers to cope with misfortunes (particularly disease).
> If Sakpata strikes a man with smallpox, it is because he
> wants to establish a very close relationship with that person.

Only the man who is not mature enough or strong enough will die of the disease. For the worthy person it is like an initiation: a death and resurrection into a maturer, [sic] richer life.[4]

Babalu is himself afflicted, usually with smallpox or leprosy, in the stories that have been spun around him. Yet in spite of his condition, he always endures, limping along accompanied by dogs-for no human companion will countenance one so hideously disfigured by illness-to become king and inherit the earth. He provides a stirring role model for all who suffer and testifies that however horrible its circumstances, life is worth living.

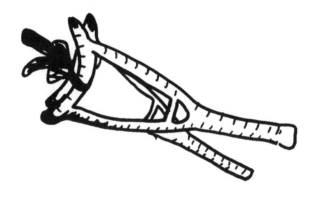

Babalu's Symbol: Crutches

2

SACRED STORIES

We know that truth about an Orisha cannot be embodied in a single narrative or viewpoint. That is because Orisha exist in cyclical time as opposed to linear time. Orisha Shango is both a primordial emanation of Olodumare generated in the sky's rage and the historic fourth emperor of the Yoruba. Multiple permutations can and usually do exist of a single Orisha. They sparkle like multiple reflections of a brilliant light in a many faceted glass. The light is no less powerful for being broken up in its display and has a profound center. Many pataki, sacred stories, explain how Babalu came to be afflicted. One is not necessarily better than any other. Fundamental truth about this Orisha is contained in each story, even if they seem to contradict one another. Such is the case in our first two pataki.

Once, Eshu Olosi, the ultimate trickster, challenged Olofi, God Almighty, to show him one righteous man that he could not tempt. He insisted that no human being could resist him. Olofi took up the gauntlet and said that Asowano was a man of such impeccable character that nothing Olosi could do would change that. Olosi laughed and asked if he could put him to a test. Olofi agreed.

Soon, Asowano's joints swelled. Ulcers erupted all over his skin. His nose caved in. His toes fell off, or maybe they were eaten by rats. One leg shriveled so, it became useless, and the once noble man now dragged himself on two crutches. He moved like a crab. Satisfied that no one would willingly endure such agony, Olosi approached him.

"You, Asowano, do you recognize me? I am Olosi, the artist of your misfortune. Just as I have made wretched, sorry little man, I can make you tall and proud once more. And all I ask of you is this, say yes to me, Olosi, sworn adversary of Olofi ...." "No," Asowano proclaimed, and dragged himself along. Olosi laughed, this would only be the beginning of the torments he devised.

Asowano hobbled through town. People threw water on him which stung his sores. "Go away, monster. Go away." Asowano looked upon them, his former friends and neighbors, and tears welled in his eyes. Yet, he refused to let his tears gush. He stiffened his hackneyed lips and bore down on his crutches. His arm muscles strained against his skin, causing ulcers to weep, and agonizingly he dragged himself away from humanity.

The hot dry sun dried the putrid smelling puss that seemed to ooze from every pore and gave scant relief. He began to favor moving around when the sun was at its peak. He settled in a grotto far removed from his village by a rustling stream. He covered the entrance with palm fibers and black cloth so that no one could see him. Dogs joined him there. They didn't seem to care how hideous or fetid he was. They tenderly licked at his sores, and strangely their tongues didn't hurt him. He grew accustomed to them. His voice had become so nasal that it almost sounded like a dog whining. Olosi presented himself again, this time with promises of great luxury in addition to healing. Asowano flailed at him with his crutch. "Go away, evil. I will have none of you! Get out. I won't change for you or for anyone." With those words, Olofi called in his marker with Olosi. "You, Olosi, have been proven wrong once and for all by a mortal. For that, I will no longer suffer your company ...." And Olosi was consigned to the lower depths, never again to approach the heaven, although he would still mingle with men.

As for Asowano, he persevered, eventually travelling to a far away land where people acknowledged him as king because of the tremendous burdens he was able to shoulder with dignity. And he became known as Obaluaye, King of the Earth.

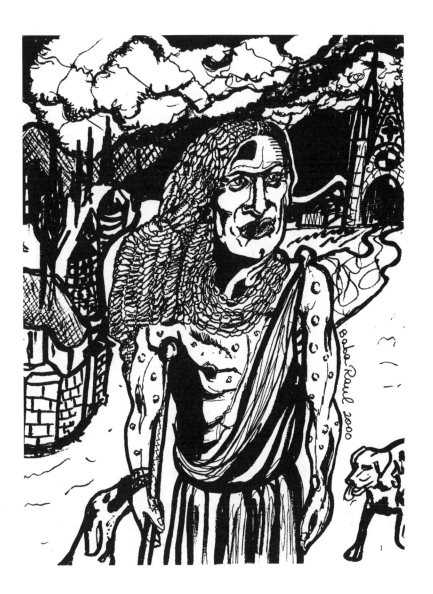

There is yet another story popularly told in Cuba about how Babalu became afflicted, and it goes like this. When Olofi distributed powers to all the different Orisha, he asked them what abilities they wanted. For Babalu, the answer was simple. He wanted fortitude as a lover to satisfy any woman at any time. Olofi agreed, but with one caveat. He had to refrain from sex just one specific day each year. Babalu agreed.

He was a happy young rake, with a lean, sinewy body, and twisted grin women found irresistible. He made ample use of his divine gift. Women began to worship him, the perpetual lover. After all, no other man could satisfy them like he could, and with such enthusiasm. Word of his exploits reached the Orisha of sensuality, Oshun. She had perfected the voluptuary arts and longed for a man who would share her joy and be able to keep up with her.

When the two met the attraction was instant. Babalu had never beheld such a woman. Maybe it was her pomegranate stained lips poised in knowing and gentle smile. Maybe the breasts molded into firm mounds with cinnamon colored tips. Or the smooth arch her hand made in the air as she batted her peacock feathered fan under inky and tremulous eyelashes. Whatever it was she had, she made him burn like no other had, Babalu knew that the instant he saw her. And even though it was the day of his appointed abstinence, the clove together and twisted themselves amidst each others perfect skin, sinew, and moist secrets.

When Oshun parted, Babalu sprawled languidly on his bed. He did not immediately perceive that Olofi had recognized his betrayal or the beginning of pocks bubbling on his physique. Within hours, the once virile man shrieked in agony. His skin had erupted so badly that it was falling in little pieces like dried beans from his bony frame. Fire that consumed him from without. A cold fist squeezed his heart from within as he realized what he had done - betray his sacred pledge to Olofi. He struggled to make his way to the archdivinity, but his legs crumpled under him as he tried to walk, and he fell upon the earth. Every inch of his skin was now encrusted with pox, and the pox became indistinguishable from the many pebbles on the ground, and that was how Babalu looked when he died. In affliction he became the scarred and pitted face of earth.

Now when Oshun heard what had happened she was horrified. Not only had Babalu been the one man who could keep reach for the same ecstatic heights as she, but his crooked smile held a certain charm like a turn in the road that leads to new vistas. She marched to Olofi's house, pounded on his door, and demanded, "Baba, what have you done to Babalu! I demand you bring him back." Olofi met her protest with silence, and Oshun thought about what she should do.

Later that night she returned to his door. She did not knock. She entered his house naked, her body glistening with honey. She reached down with her hand and gathered honey to her fingers. She quietly walked over to Olofi, who lay sleeping and smeared honey on his lips. As Olofi roused, a smile arched Oshun's pomegranate colored lips. "You want to taste more of my honey, Baba." Olofi reached for her, and as he hand stretched toward her, she drew back. "If you want to take what is mine, you have to give me something back in return..." Olofi, it would be said later, was on his knees begging for a taste of Oshun's honey. After all, it is Oshun and her abundant gifts that makes life worth living. Oshun made it clear: He would have to return Babalu to life if he was going to further taste her honey. Olofi could not refuse.

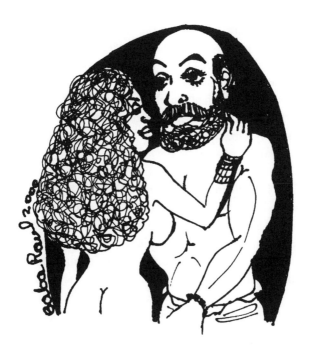

When Babalu was resurrected, he was full of the worst diseases. Syphilis flowed in his bloodstream. Leprosy bacillus hid in the cool places of his body, while smallpox virus bloomed when he heated up. Everywhere he went, pestilence became part of his stock and trade. Yet, in spite of the horror this inspired, a great dignity shone where there once had been raffish charm. Whereas once, only one damsel at a time would swoon at his virile presence, now whole nations would fall at his feet. He does not crow about this. Instead, he perseveres, and teaches those that fall at his feet that they too can be resurrected if they find strength within themselves. Dogs join him on his lonely journey until he finds a place with people strong enough to make him king.

Commentary: At first, these depictions seem incompatible. An honorable man versus a rake. Yet in both narratives, he does not compromise who he is. This defines him. Are not both the ascetic and voluptuary both wholly committed to their pursuits? Babalu never apologizes for what he does. He sticks to his guns. His is extreme clear-eyed integrity. This qualifies him to become the almighty prosecutor. Dr. Wande Abimbola points out:

> He is a very important warrior Orisa who controls the woroko. These are agents of Obaluaye [Babalu] who can wage war against people as the Ajogun can. That is why people often think Obaluaye is related to pestilence. He just doesn't go about inflicting people with smallpox or other diseases as punishment unless the person has done something for which he should be punished. When an Orisa reports to him about an evil done by someone in the community, Obaluaye will order his own warriors to punish that person.[5]

Babalu finds his way in the bush, amidst lush green shapes, perfumes of flower and fruit, insect noises and bird whistles, and peace - far away from man. His dogs sniff the earth, moving carefully ahead of his beleaguered steps. He hears someone rustles and spies a shape not far removed from his own. Hopping about with one leg, this lopsided denizen of the forest has a huge cauliflower ear popping from one side of his head, and the tiniest of holes for an ear on the other. His one eye winks at Babalu.

They sit down together on a fallen tree and laugh, recognizing how gingerly they each must negotiate this simple action. Babalu sees the other's lips moving, but the sound he hears whistles from treetops. It is not human words, yet he understands the trillings as speech. His own voice whines out from a throat coated with mucous. Again, they laugh.

As Babalu's dogs leap after tiny, quick flying things, the two realize each has very special gifts the other could find useful. Babalu controls all diseases. Osanyin, his new friend, knows all medicines - both healing and poison - contained in leaves. Between them, they could raise or fall entire civilizations at their whim. They agree to help their respective worshippers. Babalu will make people sick so Osanyin's worshippers can heal them with leaves. Thus, both Orisha would receive tribute and their devotees thrive. However, this is not how things work out.

Neither Orisha understands human greed. Soon Osanyin's children poison Babalu's, and Babalu's afflicting Osanyin's. Nobody gets well, and people turn away from worshipping either Orisha because of all the illness and bad medicine. Sitting on a fallen tree, far from humanity, both Orisha shake their heads. They make a new pact. Neither's children will hurt the other's. Hopefully, their children will do better this time.

Commentary: Babalu and Osanyin share pain of disfigurement and mysteries to achieve health and well being. As rightful owner of earth, with the help of agricultural Orisha and fellow leper, Orisha Oko, Babalu tacitly supports the leaves that grow with Osanyin's knowledge. Medicine is vital to Babalu, who must work as an itinerant, poor man's physician to help his worshippers. Ethnobotany is still the leading source for most medicines known to man. Secrets of Babalu and Osanyin must be shared to be fully understood.

The following pataki is the most often-told in Cuba about how disease entered the world. It is said that when Olodumare parcelled out portions of his power among all the Orisha, he gave Babalu the important task of guarding the sack where all diseases lay dormant. One time, during a bembe, when all of the Orisha were enjoying the drumming and the dancing, Babalu forgot that he had a slight handicap in that his left leg was shorter than his right, and began to dance the hard rhythms with abandon. Spontaneously, everyone began to laugh at him. Enraged, he let out all the dormant illnesses he had been so zealously guarding. Because of this, Olofi sent him away from Ife. He went to Dahomey, to the land of the Arara, where he became a beloved king. Since then Babalu has dedicated himself to healing those that were afflicted do to his short temper.

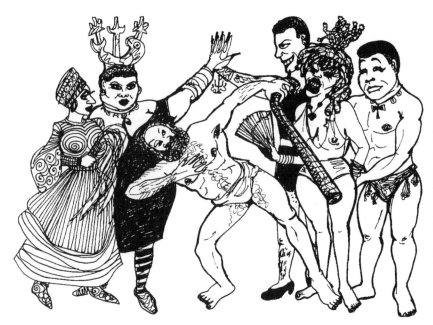

Oya, Yemoja, Inle, Oshun and Shango laugh at Babalu's attempt at dancing

Commentary: The obvious irony in this pataki is that the god of healing, Babalu, was the cause of illness coming to existence. It also emphasizes Babalu's very human qualities. He wants to take part in the rejoicing, music and dancing, but his infirmities make that impossible. The Lord giveth and the Lord taketh away, so blessed be the name of the Lord!

Another cautionary tale dealing with Babalu as Lord of Pestilence comes to us from Africa.

During the peak of the dry season, when the wind itself walked as a man in a hartaman, a plague of pox blighted Ile-Ife, the mythical birthplace of mankind. The good people of Ife stopped sweeping their houses as fevered people perforated with pustules, reminding them of a proverb about the dread one who made the grains men ate stand out on their skins. They knew Sònpònná walked in their midst.

But rather than pray to him to spare them, they sacrificed to Orunmilla to deliver them, and thus a surreal battle of titans ensued. Orunmilla set out to meet the provocateur head on, and Sònpònná with two hundred flames shooting from his head met him. Shocked at such a fearsome sight, Orunmilla withdrew. Then he sucked up all the water in Ife and spat on Sònpònná to put out his fire. Sonponna charged Orunmilla and engaged him in hand to hand combat. Again Orunmilla withdrew, and this time he ate all the crops in Ife to gather strength so that he could bare down on Sònpònná. But rather than recoil, Sònpònná hurled poison arrows at Orunmilla. Now Orunmilla grabbed people to shield himself from Sònpònná's onslaught. Sònpònná spent his last arrow. Orunmilla began eating people to gather up strength for one final charge with which he finally repelled Sònpònná.

Finished with this harrowing ordeal, Orunmilla went back to the people of Ife expecting tribute. Instead he met the few people left with looks of horror etched into their faces. "Orunmilla, what have you done to us?" they cried out. "We asked you to save of us from Sònpònná's affliction, and instead you devastated us worse than he ever has."

Commentary: This pataki reminds us of the age-old adage: sometimes the cure is worse than the disease. Diseases test our mettle. Often our bodies and souls find resources to stand up to their challenge. Medicines often have severe consequences themselves. Constant use of antibiotics has been proven to create stronger treatment-resistant pathogens. Many of the sophisticated drug cocktails used to curb HIV-infection have now been shown to have severe side effects, such as disfigurement, osteoporosis, bone marrow depletion and compromised organ systems. This is not an argument to avoid medical treatment of HIV or any other malady, rather a reminder that we need to weigh our options. Also, the people of Ife failed to honor Babalu. By turning to Orunmilla for help with something that was Babalu's rightful province, they inadvertently made their situation much worse.

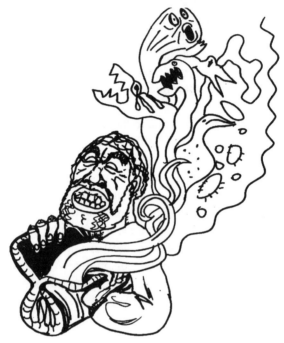

Babaluaye unleashes pestilence upon the world

Yet another African tale recorded by Ulli Beier reminds us about universal truths about justice.

Once there was a prosperous man, Babaniyangi, who had five sons: Ogun, Eshu, Orisha Oko, Shango, Orunmilla and Sònpònná. When he passed away, his children followed him to heaven to make appropriate funeral tribute. Once their obligations were met, they returned to earth. On their way, they stopped to rest under an Iroko tree. Sònpònná, the youngest, kindly volunteered to go fetch water for his older siblings. When he was away, the four greedily divided their father's belongings, completely forsaking the youngest.

When Sònpònná returned, he asked what had become of his share. His brothers told him that they had forgotten him. He stormed away in anger, but Orunmilla stopped him. He told him that he would get his just due if he returned to heaven. There he would find a bow, arrow, stick and string. Sònpònná returned to earth with these, and Orunmilla told him to seek the services of one of his apprentice diviners. The diviner told the young man that he would become more powerful than all his brothers if he made sacrifice. After completing the instructions he was given, Sònpònná prayed at his father's grave. His father spoke to him: "You, my son, will have the nations of this world bow down to you. I will tell you a secret incantation. Use it and you shall overcome your brothers and all men."

Sònpònná on his return to earth shot arrows to the four corners and repeated his father's incantation. Smallpox came into the world and felled men everywhere. In the land of Sònpònná's birth, people pleaded with Orunmilla to divine the cause of this plague. Orunmilla revealed that he and his brothers had betrayed their youngest brother, and that the young man's search for justice had brought disease into the world. He advised people to sacrifice to Sònpònná and ask his forgiveness.

People everywhere began to worship Sònpònná, and the outbreak of smallpox stopped. Sònpònná became known as Obaluaye, King of the Earth.

Commentary: Here, we are reminded of the need to treat everyone fairly. Babalu's outrage is just. When he is given justice, he no longer strikes out at anyone with pestilence.

3

ATTRIBUTES

Necklace:

Babalu's necklace typically consists of white beads striped with blue. However, each of his roads has its own specific beading patterns.

Shrine (igbodu) How initiates honor Babalu

Babalu is not usually "made" in Santería, though he is in Arará and in Candomble. This means he is not presented to the head but is given so that he may be an integral presence in someone's life. It is usually indicated in a reading of cowries if he needs to be vested, often it is for reasons of health or economic well being. One need not be a priest of Santeria in order to get Babalu.

Babalu's mysteries are kept inside a clay or porcelain pot covered with a piece of burlap and cowries. Inside are two iron dogs, 18 cowries, and 7 pieces of coral or reef stone. The use of coral rather than stones is particularly significant. The scaly appearance of coral mimics many of the skin diseases governed by Babalu. Also, corals are composed of thousands of tiny animals, just as a infections are composed of vast number of bacteria or virus. Beside the pot are a pair of crutches and a ja.

A ja (pronounced "ha") is a broom of fibers used in cleansings. It is made up of a makuto (medicine bag) containing coconut fibers, seven guinea peppers, a piece of tiger skin, and herbs sacred to Babalu. These ingredients are mashed together and rolled up in a piece of red cloth, which is overlaid with sackcloth and sewn shut. This along with a cockspur is hidden inside. The broom is adorned with two rows of sixteen cowry shells and beads patterned to the specific path of Babalu. (Note: a ja can be given separately. It can only be made by a bona fide priest, one who has received Babalu.) Babalu is accompanied by his mother, Nana Bukuu, and his own Elegua, Afra - who unlike other Eleguas comes as a piece of brain coral in his own herb pot. (Note: Afra does not take rum and may punish those who offer it to him with a nasty rash.)

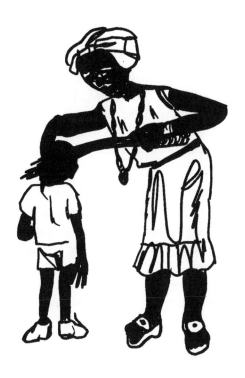

Healing with Babalu's "JA"

Making Babalu

Rarely does anyone have Orisha Babalu crowned to his head in Santeria, although he is still frequently crowned in Santeria's sister religion in Brazil, Candomble, and in Arara (Cuban-Dahomeyan religion).

Shrine (olujo alejo) How non-initiates may begin to honor Babalu

Babalu may be honored with a simple shrine to reflect his humble tastes. Appropriate objects include sack cloth, raffia, straw, brooms, dry grains, sesame flowers, representations of dogs, crutches and San Lazaro statues and chromoliths. Non-initiates may wear a cacha, a bracelet of goat skin and cowries on their left wrist to symbolize their devotion to Babalu.

Blood Offerings (ebo):

Traditionally, Babalu takes guinea hen, old castrated goat, and occasionally speckled pigeon.

Offerings (adimu):

The standard offering for Babalu is a bottle of dry white wine, sesame seed, a bowl of milk and bread (for his dogs.) He also likes dried beans of many colors, grains, toasted corn and tobacco. Do not include water in any offering to Babalu. In fact his omiero is made with green coconut milk or dry white wine. (Water irritates his sores.)

Characteristics of Babalu (and of his devotees):

Babalu's Catholic disguise is St. Lazarus. This is not the Lazarus whom Christ rose from the dead. Rather he is the beggar referred to in the parable that it is easier to pass through the eye of a needle than for a rich man to get into heaven.

The dramatic story of the rich man and the beggar occurs in Luke, xvi, 19-31:

> **Their Condition Here:** The rich man was clothed in purple and byssus (D.V. fine linen), and spent each day in gay carousing. The beggar had been cast helpless at the rich man's gate, and lay there all covered with sores; he yearned for the crumbs that fell from the rich man's table, but received none, and was left to the dogs.

Their Condition Hereafter: The early banquet is over; the heavenly banquet is begun. Lazarus partakes of the banquet in a place of honor (cf. John, xiii, 23). He reclines his head on Abraham's bosom. The rich man is now the outcast. He yearns for a drop of water. Lazarus is not allowed to leave the heavenly banquet and tend to the outcast.

Like Babalu, St. Lazarus is depicted as a leper, and became a special intercessor for lepers and all the afflicted during the Middle Ages. His feast day in Cuba is celebrated on December 17th. Of all the Saints used to disguise Yoruba Orisha, the identification of Lazaro with Babalu runs deeper than any. Even Santeros of many years, who would never dream of referring to Shango as "St. Barbara" or Yemaya as "Regla," will still call Babalu San Lazaro.

Babalu's colors are purple, gold and, in Africa, scarlet. His numbers are eleven, thirteen and seventeen. When eleven shells fall face up in the Dilogun oracle, it is called "Ojuani," where Babalu speaks, and the accompanying refrain is " you, can't carry water in a basket." According to Judith Gleason, this odu (known in Africa as Owonrin): "is an extremely dangerous sign: an indication of persistent drought, famine, and lingering disease, all conditions associated with Babaluaye...son of outraged earth that refuses to yield, and a the dry wind that brings premonitions of epidermal and abdominal maladies."[6] It is in Ojuani Meji that Babalu undergoes his ordeals yet becomes King. When 13 shells speak in Dilogun, it is called Metanla, where the proverb says "Where illness is born, blood is bad." Here too lies Babalu's domain. In the African telling of this Odu (which is named Ika in Africa) Babalu is horribly scarred by negligence of elders who use unclean knives to give him his tribal facial marks. His outrage over his disfigurement and their irresponsibility brings pestilence into the world. It is an odu associated with revenge, manipulation and control. Babalu's association with the number seventeen has two sources: St. Lazarus' holy day and that he has seventeen distinct paths in Africa.

Babalu is the patron Orisha of anyone who is afflicted with a contagious disease. Babalu also protects the poor and those who suffer unjustly. He is God's prosecutor who afflicts the unjust and liars with both pestilence and mental illness. In Africa, he rides as a warrior on a mule, carrying a bag of poison-tipped arrows. In the New World he is an itinerant on crutches accompanied by dogs. His children as those born with Babalu on their heads are called, tend to be serious loners. Those who remember priests of Babalu from Cuba, often describe them as having been disfigured, such as one bearing leprosy scars or having suffered an amputation. Often they are marked by numerous birth marks or scars. They are often born healers who live with maladies themselves. Children of Babalu must abstain from eating sesame and lentils, because lentils remind the Orisha of his leprosy.

Lydia Cabrera states that Babalu's messengers are mosquitoes and flies.[7] This is tied up to his role as bringer of pestilence, since these two pests are notorious carriers of disease.

Herbs and plants:

Cundiamor (a.k.a bitter melon), wormwood, peppermint, wild tobacco, sesame, cactus, palm fronds, chives, and akoko leaves.

ROADS OF BABALU AND THEIR BEADS:

Asoyin: an Arara path, "Father of the Rain that Kills with Burning temperatures": He kills with smallpox. 17 brown beads, 3 black, 1 azabache, 3 blacks, 17 browns until the desired length.

Nana Buruku: Sometimes thought to be a female path of Babalu, or his mother. In our house, we always give Nana and Afra at the same time we give Babalu. Necklace: Eleven black beads with one azabache until desired length is reached.

Ayanó: Necklace: 17 white with blue stripes (henceforth called "Babalu beads"), 7 red, until desired length is reached.

Awo: 17 Babalu beads, 3 black beads, I azabache (jet) bead, plus 3 black, 17 Babalu beads, etc.

Afimayé: A gravedigger, this path walks with Oya. Necklace: 11 Babalu beads, nine brown etc.

Álua: Wisdom personified. 17 black, 1 azabache.

Baba Arúgbo or Aribo: Ancient Father. 7 brown beads, 1 black, 1 brown, and so on.

Aliprete: 17 blue, 3 black, 1 azabache, 3 black, 17 Babalu beads, until desired length is reached.

Shakpata, Shoppono: Small pox personified: 11 dark blue, 11 Babalu beads, one azabache, etc.

Lokuon: 17 brown, 7 brown with white stripes (Oya beads), etc.

Azudo: 13 or 17 black, 7 brown, and so on.

Other roads of Babalu: Suju, Dakunambo, Afrekete, Kake, and Usunike. In Palo he is called Kubayende and Pata-en Llaga.

Roads in Africa: According to Karin Barber, in her seminal Article "How man makes god in West Africa: Yoruba Attitudes toward the Orisa, Africa, Vol. 51 No. 31981, p. 732, Babalu has seventeen "designations" in Yorubaland, including:

Waríwarùn: A staunch defender of his devotees who' instantly possesses them when they are beaten.

Àbàtà: Literally, "swamp," he cannot stand the noise made by scraping a cooking pot.

Adégbònà: He cannot be splashed with water

Ògáálá: He uses a tiny branding iron to make smallpox scars on people.

Babalu in Brazil:

Also syncretized with St. Lazarus, Orixa Omolú holds a position in Afro-Brazilian religions as important as he does in Cuba. One Brazilian legend holds that his mother, Nana abandoned him as a baby because he was colicky. Left by the ocean's edge, crabs descended on the helpless infant eating away his face and crippling him. Yemanja rescued him and raised him as her own. Still, when he is evoked, his true mother Nana is almost always included. His sister /brother is the rainbow serpent Oshumare. Sometimes his horses wear snakes as laurels in their hair. His province is illness. He appears covered in straw, with a straw mask that forms a pointed cone, to cover his disfigurement. His implement is the ñàñàrà- a bundle of palm fronds (igi öpë) decorated with Cowries - similar to a ja. His colors are red, black, and white, and his day is Monday.

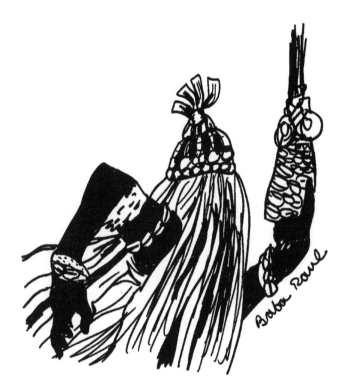

Omolú (Brazilian Babalu)

4

BABALÚ AND SANTERÍA'S "CELESTIAL COURT"

As the spirit of healing, Babalu is an Orisha of enormous importance. His mother is Nana Bukuu, who is the primordial mother embodied by the moon and swamp. She always partakes of Babalu's offerings, as does his Elegua, Afra. His sister/brother is Oshumaré, the rainbow serpent.

Many of Babalu's traditions among Santeria practitioners have been filtered through one of Cuba's other Afro-Cuban religions, Arara. Arara evolved from the Fon and the Evhe who were also brought to Cuba as salves. They worship a pantheon of deities, called fodus, that are interchangeable with Orisha. As Asoyi, Babalu is king of the Arara, and occupies the central position in their pantheon.

Among Orisha, Babalu's okinrini, one heart, is Shango. Shango befriended him in exile and stole the dogs from Ogun to provide Babalu with companionship. Therefore, Shango eats first when Babalu is to be crowned, and a Babalu priest does not attack Shango's children.

Although in Santeria hagiography Babalu is known to strike with the most terrible ailments, it is his own ability to live with affliction that gives hope to devotees whatever odds they face. Babalu is rightful owner of earth. Disease symbolizes earth's ultimate dominion over humanity. It brings human's face to face with earth through death and burial. Also, soil harbors a wide variety of infectious microbes.

Babalu lives apart from the other Orisha. In the Celestial court he is thought of as both pariah and indispensable king. During bembes, drum feast for the Orisha, water is poured on the ground when Babalu's song is first played. Devotees anoint themselves with water so that Babalu will not visit the festivities with contagion.

Although possession by Babalu rarely happens, when it does it is a dramatic event. According to Julio Garcia Cortez in his well known book, *The Osha:*

> "His trances are the most dramatic of all trances given by any Orisha. It is characterized by a tightening of the muscles, foaming at the mouth, twisting his hands and legs, while the face becomes very tense. He-she will contort for a long time eventually falling to the ground in what could easily be mistaken for an epileptic fit."

Highly feared in Africa, in Cuba his kinder aspects as a lover and a healer are emphasized, so that he is the most beloved of all Orisha. Although Shango may be the most admired and Oshun the most invoked, It is "the Old Man" who inspires the most tender feelings in Cuba. Babalu's place in Santeria's Celestial Court is paramount in an unusual way, for although he is called "el santo mayor" (the greatest of all) he is also held in awe because of his capacity to inflict dreaded diseases. While he teaches some of life's harder lessons, he generously aids believers in getting through them.

5

DESPOJOS
CLEANSINGS WITH BABALÚ

Stability and Economic Well-being:

A very popular cleansing with Babalu involves buying a bag of seven bean soup mix. Place the mixture inside an empty gourd. Next to it goes another gourd placed on a blue cloth. Ritualistically take two handfuls of beans from the calabash and pass them over your body. Then empty the beans into the other calabash. All the time you are doing this, pray to Babalu to bring you stability and economic well being. Continue with this procedure each day until the beans have completely changed gourds three times. At the end of seventeen days, wrap the beans in the cloth, cleanse your body with it one more time then take it along with seventeen cents to the woods.

Money Drawing:

A popular offering for money requires 7 roasted cobs of corn and 7 bread rolls. Place them on a white plate for seven days in front of a lit 7-day candle for Babalu. At the end of the week, take these to the woods with seventeen cents.

For treating illness:

To treat skin ailments, offer a piece of bread to Babalu, then use that same piece as a sponge, putting palm oil directly on the affected area with it.

For treating a disease:

Place an statue of St. Lazarus on an altar. Wipe the person afflicted or yourself with purple cloth and sack cloth, then drape these around the Lazarus icon. Then rub any skin eruptions with purple onions. Place the onions around a plate of grains. Light a seven day purple or yellow candle. Each morning and night pray to Babalu asking him for help healing. When the onions rot, take them, the grains and cloth, and bury them beside a river, thanking Babalu for his intercession.

For Good Luck:

Nail a piece of bread tied with a purple ribbon behind your door for good luck.

Keep Away Evil:

To keep away evil, mix sesame seeds with palm oil, mercury, and black pepper kernels (7). Offer to Babalu, asking him for protection and health.

Babalu reveals a cure for insect bites to Eric:

Whenever I work with herbs, I follow the three principles taught by my elders: 1) Only accept or buy herbs from a reliable, reputable, source. 2) Verify that the herb is non-toxic. 3) Confirm any herb prescribed in a dream through both divination and medical resources.

My first experience in healing another person with the help of Babalu occured when Michael Lemmon, a member of the Orisha Consciousness Movement and a free-lance writer, came to interview me for a local (Baltimore) newspaper. After the interview, he tells me that a spider bit him in his thigh three weeks before, and the bite won't heal, indeed, it is getting worse. I examine it. It's about the size of a golf ball, red in color, and very hard to the touch. It does not weep or yield pus when pressed.

I suggest we talk to Babalu about it after we take a walk down by the pier in Fells Point (a touristy part of Baltimore). Shortly after we begin our walk, we come across a beggar. He walks painfully with two crutches; both legs are bandaged with stained gauze. His face is marked with open sores. I immediately reach into my pockets and give him all my money--about a dollar in change. I ask him if he wants cigarettes. He says "yes," he seems embarrassed when I give him a pack. I tell him not to worry, I understand. If he'd had a dog with him, I would have prayed to him!

I tell Michael that meeting the beggar is an explicit sign that we need to take the matter of his ailment to Babalu. When we get home, we open the cabinet in which Babalu resides. I keep consecrated pieces of coconut nearby for divinatory purposes. I ask Babalu if he wishes to help Michael with his ailment, he says yes.

I proceed to ask specific questions about how to treat Michael's injury. I confirm each part of the prescription with a second throw to make sure I have the orisha's affirmation. The prescription follows: 1) Clean the bite with dry white wine and apply a compress of the same overnight; 2) Drink bitter melon (Momordica balsdamina) tea for seven consecutive nights; 3) Erect an altar to Nana Bukuu with a picture of Our Lady of Mount Carmel, burlap, and raffia; 4) light a yellow seven-day candle to Nana; 5) pass a handful of mixed beans over the injury daily for seven days and then dispose of them at least three blocks away from home; 6) be confident Nana and Babalu will heal you. I also confirm the total prescription by throwing the coconut oracle again.

After five days, Michael calls excitedly to say his injury has healed! I tell him to continue with the plan anyway, to make sure it doesn't return.

Bitter melon tea

Since then, under the wise guidance of Baba Raul, I have learned to work with this wonderful force we call Babalu. Babalu has become my very special friend. His most striking healing plant is bitter melon, called cundiamor in Cuba. I was meditating on Babalu in front of his shrine one day when a local African-based priestess of Ogun called to tell me that she had come across some cundiamor and wanted to share it with me. I hadn't yet become familiar with the plant, so she tells me some basics about it. Used in spiritual baths, it dispells negative vibrations and helps clear blemishes. Ingested as a tea, it detoxifies. Many years ago, Baba had a revelation from Babalu instructing him to treat his godchildren with AIDS with bitter melon tea. Recent scientific research bears out the wisdom of may wish to mix it with spearmint because it tastes so bitter!

I wait until a day when I ache all over and I am overwhelmed by fatigue. I crumble both leaves and stalk into a cup of water and boil it, then strain out the vegetable matter. The tea smalls nice, like Earl Gray, but the taste is horrible, like chewing on aspirin. I drink the tea nonetheless and find myself pain-free and energized within half an hour! I have a dream that night where Babalu instructs me on the qualities of cundiamor. It has antiviral properties akin to antioxidants and can be used to improve immune function.

Healing acne

Boil one cup of rice in three cups of water until rice has consistency of grits. Add one teaspoonful of almond oil. Pray to Babalu that he may bless your efforts. Let rice paste cool to slightly above room temperature, apply like a mask, let it stay on your face for about one hour, remove and wash your face with water. Repeat daily until acne clears up.

Healing hemorrhoids

Carefully pass a needle and strong thread through seven cashew nuts, preferably raw. Let each nut be about four inches away from each other. Wear cashews around your waist, under your outer clothes, until problematic hemorrhoids get better.

Seeking Babalu's intervention in surgery

Promise Babalu you'll give him a likeness in solid gold of whatever you are going to have operated if you come out OK. After the surgery, have the gold charm in the form of a leg, a liver, or whatever ready to be presented to a statue of St. Lazarus in a church, or a Babalu deity in a Santero's shrine. As we have said, Cuba's main St. Lazarus shrine at El Rincon is covered with hundreds of thousands of dollars worth of gold legs, arms, hearts, livers, and all kinds of body organs from thousands upon thousands of grateful suppliants.

All-around good luck Babalu cleansing:

Buy seven different kinds of dried beans, for example, navy, lima, pink, kidney, chick peas, split peas, and lentils. Each morning, make a little packet with one kind of bean for each member of your family, instructing them to carry them around with them all day, later throwing it away at night. At the end of the seven days, light a yellow candle thanking Babalu for his blessings.

Babalu unhexing bath:

Take three teaspoons of sesame oil, three drops of patchouli oil, and three drops of honey. Add to bathwater. Light purple candle to Babalu, while taking bath, repeat the following:

> *"Oh blessed Babalu, you who conquered disease to become king, break whatever evil, from within or without, is keeping me from success. Amen, Amen, Amen."*

Babalu bath to attract a lover of the opposite sex:

Boil 12 pumpkin seeds in a quart of water, two tablespoons of honey, a pinch of salt, a bunch of spearmint, and one bay leaf. Strain, pouring liquid into bathwater. If you are a man, say the following:

> *"You were **chulo** as well as king, take me please under your wing. As the **mamis** took to thee, let them also come to me."*

Women should say:

> *"You were **chulo** as well as king, take me please under your wing. As the **mamis** took to thee, let the **papis** come to me."*

Within seven days, you'll notice a marked improvement in your love life. This spell was developed by the famed Louisiana Voodoo king Dr. John.

Mae Rabanito's Omolu money-drawing bath:

Make a pot full of lentil soup, feed it to dogs. Light a green candle to Omolu (Brazilian name for Babalu), asking him to give you the blessings of money. After you get the money, give Omolu a solid gold dollar sign as thanks.

Babalu unhexing, good luck floor wash:

Take 17 bay leaves, a bunch of bitter melon leaves, corn husks, and sesame oil. Mix with bucket of water, wash floors, beginning in the back, ending in the front.

Fertility spell for barren women:

Take a bitter melon fruit, annoint with honey, place in front of lit yellow seven-day candle for thirty minutes. Pray to Babalu for fertility. Touch honey-covered fruit to your vagina. Wrap in yellow cloth, leave in garbage can at a maternity ward or hospital. Make love every night while candle is burning, you'll get pregnant.

To make a bone heal fast:

Take a bone from a chicken's leg, tie a purple ribbon around it until it is almost totally covered with it, light a purple seven-day candle on the new moon at 2:00 A.M. and place the chicken bone in front of the candle, when the candle is spent, place bone, wax remains from candle, and some sesame seeds along with seven pennies inside a small paper bag. Throw away in a garbage far from home. Annoint the affected part (leg, arm, or whatever) with a mixture of patchouli, almond, and mineral oil. Wrap with ace bandage, if possible. Give Babalu 17 yellow roses when the break heals.

To make two people fight:

Write names of the two people you want to see fighting on two separate pieces of a brown paper bag. Get a piece of raw meat, add vinegar, chili, onions, whole pepper kernels, lime juice, and garlic to it. Feed to a mean dog, such as a pit bull.

Invoking Babalu (per Maria-José):

According to Brazilian priestess Mae Maria-José, as reported by Serge Bramly in his book Macumba (City Lights: San Francisco, 1994), you can invoke Omulu's protection by reciting the following with great faith:

> *"Omulu, hear your child! You have the strength, the strength a child needs! Come to his aid! You are old but you are wise and powerful!"*

You can also keep Babalu's protection always with you by drawing the following sygill with dragon's blood ink on parchment and saving it on a little leather bag you can always carry, or wear as a pendant.

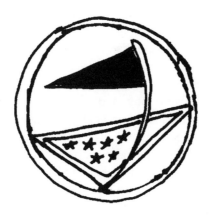

6

Oriki Babalú / Orin Babalú
Prayers and Songs to Babalú

In Cuba, it is said that when we talk to the Orisha in their own language, it makes them better disposed to grant our petition. Priesthood holders are expected to learn the songs and praises to the Orisha in Lukumi, an archaic form of Yoruba that developed in Cuba. Because Yoruba is a tonal language, and in Cuba the Lukumi did not develop a system of writing down the different tonalities, Lukumi songs and prayers are often hard to render into standard Yoruba. John Mason, a priest of Obatala operating out of Brooklyn, New York, has dedicated a great deal of time and effort to render Lukumi songs into standard Yoruba, a laudable effort. Add to that the fact that the Yoruba love to pun, and you find yourself with a very hard task when trying to decipher these songs. The effort we make in trying to sing these praises to our beloved Orisha, however, does not go unnoticed by them. I think the Orisha must be pleased that we are at least trying!

ORIN BABALU

Baba e, Baba soro só
Lord father, fierce [and] dogged
Baba e, Baba soro só
Lord father, fierce [and] dogged
Babalúaiyé iyan ko'mo'de
Father of the World, famine, no-son-crown
Baba s'iré siré
Father give us blessings, give us blessings

Lord Father, Fierce and Dogged
Lord Father, Fierce and Dogged
Lord Father of the World and Famine,
King without Heir Give us great blessings!

ORIKI BABALU (ARARÁ)

Asoyin, fodu potente, rey del mundo
Arara Yo so' omo' osi Afrekete,
ma' si omo, Afrekete no fuera,
de to tierra yo quisiera.
Mai'se'bo, mai' se' bo,
dame to que to pedi, mai'se'bo.

Babalu (Asoyin), potent god.
King of the world, king of the Arara.
I am a child of Yemaya (Afrekete),
yet if I were not a child of Yemaya,
from your land I'd like to be.
I've offered you sacrifice, I've offered you sacrifice,
now grant my wish, for I've offered you sacrifice.

ORIKI BABALU
(Translated from Lukumi by Yeyita Garcia)

Gbogbo enla nisun wonkoyi
Sonpona dakun yimini yara-mi
Sonpona ile mi bumi,
A lile mi bumi kowo
ibariba lile mi bumi
Alile mi bumi kowo
Engo begun gun-gun
Daiku Madari oro si elewa
Sonpona korisigbo
O ran moleru korisigbo

Everyone's in a deep, wakeless sleep
Babalu, wake me in my sleeping chamber
Babalu, pass over my hut.
It would be bad for you not to pass over my hut.
Father of Fathers, pass over my hut.
It would be bad for you not to pass over my hut.
I will follow the egun to their place of rest.
Laughter in the hut, handsome one laughs.
Trickster bring money to my hut.
Babalu go to the forest.
You are the one who helps men carry their loads to the forest.

ORIKI BABALU

Iso Aparo	Partridge fart
Rira n'Iso aparo ra	The partridge fart is lost
Iso aparo	Partridge fart
Rira n'Iso aparo ra	The partridge fart is lost
Ti o nso enia di talaka	To make someone loose his property.[8]

ORIN BABALU (per John Mason)

Gbogbo ènia ni nsùn ti won kò ji,
Sònponná, dákun ji mi ni yàrá mi,
Sònponná, f'ilé mi bun mi,
Ìbàribà f'ilé mi bun mi.
Ai f'ilé mi bun mi ko wo.
Ngo b'egún Ngo b'egun re'lé,
Tere tere'gun, gùn gùn
Daiko, Má da'ri orb s'ile wa.
Sònponná, kori s'igbó,
O ran 'mo Peru ko ri s'igbó.

All people sleep and never awake,
Babalu, please wake me up in my room,
Babalu spare me my house,
It is bad if you do not spare my house.
Ibariba (Babalu) spare me my house.
It is bad if you do not spare my house.
I will follow the ancestors, follow the ancestors home,
Happy, Happy, Happy home
Masquerader divert wealth into our house
Babalu go in the bush,
You are the one who when helping someone to carry his
burden, carries it into the bush.[9]

[1] Ulli Beier, Yoruba Poetry (Cambridge, Great Britain: Cambridge University Press, 1970), pp.29-30.

[2] Although the African spelling of this word is "Aiye," I am rendering it here as it has been spelled in Cuban Santeria for hundreds of years. B.R.C.

[3] John Mason, Orin Orisha (New York: Yoruba Theological Archministry, 1992), p.160.

[4] Ulli Beier, Yoruba myths (Cambridge: Cambridge University Press, 1980), p.76.

[5] Wande Abimbola, Ifa Will Mend Our Broken World (Roxbury, MA: AIM Books, 1997), p. 122.

[6] Judith Gleason, A Recitation of Ifa (New York: Grossman, 1973), p. 97.

[7] Lydia Cabrera, El Monte (Miami: Ediciones Universal, 1986), p.49.

[8] Pierre Fatunmbi Verger, Awon EweOsanyin-Yoruba Medicinal Leaves (Ile Ife: Institute of African Studies, 1967), p.50.

[9] John Mason, Orin Orisa: Songs for Selected Heads (Brooklyn, New York: Yoruba Theological Archministry, 1992), p. 138.

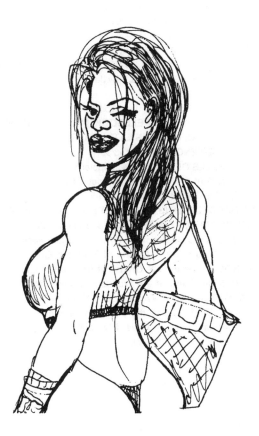